Fix Your Hormones and Fix Your Weight

A Step-by-Step Guide to Resetting Your Hormones and Sustainable Fat Loss

By Jasmin Brooks

Introduction

Are you tired of struggling with diets that leave you feeling deprived and discouraged? Are you ready to unlock the secrets to weight loss that lasts—without extreme restrictions, exhausting workouts, or quick-fix promises that never work?

Fix Your Hormones and Fix Your Weight offers a breakthrough approach that goes beyond calorie-counting and meal plans, targeting the real root of weight struggles: your hormones. In this practical, science-backed guide, you'll discover how rebalancing key hormones like insulin, cortisol, thyroid, and sex hormones can help you achieve sustainable weight loss, renewed energy, and a sense of well-being that feels effortless.

In this book, you'll learn how to:

- **Identify and correct hormonal imbalances** that lead to weight gain, cravings, and fatigue.

- **Eat for hormonal health** with a balanced, satisfying approach that stabilizes your blood sugar, boosts your metabolism, and keeps you full of energy.

- **Manage stress and improve sleep quality** to support cortisol balance and reduce weight-gain triggers.

- **Design a personalized exercise plan** that supports your hormones and your weight goals, without over-stressing your body.

- **Avoid common environmental toxins** that disrupt hormones, and adopt simple habits to create a hormone-friendly lifestyle.

Complete with self-assessment tools, customizable meal plans, and tips for sustainable lifestyle shifts, **Fix Your Hormones and Fix Your Weight** is the ultimate guide to creating a life that supports your goals for the long term. Whether you're battling stubborn belly fat, navigating weight fluctuations, or simply seeking a more holistic way to stay fit, this book will empower you with the tools to build a balanced body and a confident, healthy life.

If you're ready to break free from diet culture and discover a way to feel lighter, stronger, and more energized than ever, **Fix Your Hormones and Fix Your Weight** is your key to a healthier future. Embrace the power of hormonal health and experience the life-changing transformation you deserve!

Content:

Chapter 1

The Hormone-Weight Connection

In our pursuit of weight loss, we often focus on diet, exercise, and calorie counts. Yet, for many people, these efforts alone don't bring the lasting results they're after. This chapter will explore a crucial and often overlooked factor: **hormones**. Understanding how hormonal imbalances impact weight is essential to achieving meaningful, sustainable changes in your body. Hormones are like messengers that control nearly every function in your body, including your metabolism, appetite, mood, and energy levels. When they're in balance, your body operates efficiently. But when they're out of balance, they can lead to weight gain, fatigue, and a host of other issues.

What Are Hormones, and Why Do They Matter for Weight?

Hormones are chemical messengers produced by glands in your endocrine system. They travel through your bloodstream to organs and tissues, instructing them on what to do and when to do it.

Think of them as traffic signals directing the flow of biochemical information throughout your body. Hormones regulate critical functions like:

- **Metabolism** – the process of turning food into energy.
- **Appetite and Satiety** – signals that control hunger and fullness.
- **Fat Storage** – determining where and how much fat your body stores.
- **Mood and Energy Levels** – affecting your motivation, resilience, and stress response.

When these processes are working well, it's easier to lose weight, keep it off, and maintain good energy levels. However, various lifestyle factors—including poor diet, stress, lack of sleep, and exposure to toxins—can throw hormones out of balance, leading to unwanted weight gain and difficulty losing weight. Conventional diets often ignore these hormonal factors, focusing only on calories in and calories out. This narrow view overlooks the underlying cause of weight gain for many people: a hormonal imbalance.

Why Conventional Diets Fail Without Addressing Hormones

Conventional diets usually focus on caloric restriction and temporary eating plans that aren't sustainable. While calorie control is part of weight loss, it's not the full story. When you restrict calories without considering your hormones, several things can go wrong:

- **Hormonal Rebound**: Severe calorie restriction can cause stress on the body, leading to a rise in cortisol levels. This stress hormone triggers fat storage, particularly in the abdominal area. High cortisol can also increase cravings for high-sugar, high-fat foods, making it challenging to stick to a restrictive diet.

- **Slowed Metabolism**: When you cut too many calories, your body may respond by slowing down your metabolism to conserve energy. This process, controlled largely by thyroid hormones, can make it harder to lose weight and easier to gain it back once the diet ends.

- **Increased Hunger Hormones**: Calorie-restrictive diets can increase levels of ghrelin, the hormone that makes you feel hungry, while reducing leptin, the hormone that signals fullness. This imbalance leads to increased appetite and cravings, making it hard to sustain weight loss.

- **Unsustainable Lifestyle**: Diets that don't address the hormonal drivers of hunger, energy, and mood tend to be hard to maintain. When weight loss feels like a constant uphill battle, it's easy to give up.

To lose weight effectively and keep it off, it's essential to consider how hormones influence your body's responses to food, exercise, and lifestyle choices. This approach goes beyond calorie counting to target the root causes of weight gain.

Key Hormones That Influence Weight

There are several hormones directly involved in weight management. Here's a quick overview of the primary hormones you'll encounter in this book and how they influence your body's ability to lose or gain weight.

- **Insulin**: Often known as the "storage hormone," insulin regulates blood sugar by helping cells absorb glucose for energy. When insulin levels are balanced, your body efficiently uses glucose as fuel. However, consistently high insulin levels (often due to a diet high in sugar and refined carbs) can lead to insulin resistance. In this state, your body struggles to use glucose properly, leading to fat storage, particularly around the abdomen, and making weight loss difficult.

- **Cortisol**: Known as the "stress hormone," cortisol helps regulate energy during stressful situations. When you experience stress—whether from life pressures, poor diet, or lack of sleep—your body releases cortisol, which prompts it to store fat, especially visceral fat around the belly. Chronically elevated cortisol levels can lead to increased appetite, cravings for sugary and fatty foods, and difficulties with weight management.

- **Thyroid Hormones** (T3 and T4): The thyroid gland produces hormones that are essential for metabolism and energy regulation. When your thyroid is underactive (hypothyroidism), your metabolism slows down, leading to fatigue and weight gain. Conversely, an overactive thyroid (hyperthyroidism) can cause weight loss, though it is less common. Supporting thyroid health through proper diet, stress management, and reducing exposure to toxins can be key to maintaining a healthy metabolism.

- **Leptin and Ghrelin**: Leptin and ghrelin are known as "hunger hormones." Leptin is produced by fat cells and signals fullness to the brain, while ghrelin, produced in the stomach, signals hunger. In individuals with excess weight, leptin levels are often high, but the brain doesn't respond to it correctly—this is known as leptin resistance. Meanwhile, ghrelin levels can increase when we restrict calories or skip meals, leading to stronger hunger signals. Balancing these hormones is crucial for controlling appetite and achieving long-term weight management.

- **Sex Hormones** (Estrogen and Testosterone): Estrogen and testosterone play significant roles in body composition and fat distribution. In women, estrogen levels that are too high or too low can lead to weight gain, particularly in the hips, thighs, and abdomen. Testosterone, more dominant in men, affects muscle mass and fat distribution. When levels are low, it can lead to increased body fat and reduced muscle mass. Balancing sex hormones is important for both men and women to maintain a healthy weight and body composition.

By understanding the hormone-weight connection, you're taking the first critical step toward a new approach to weight loss—one that doesn't rely on willpower alone but works with your body's natural signals. In the following chapters, we'll dive deeper into each of these hormones and provide you with tools to balance them, enabling you to achieve lasting weight loss and a healthy body for the long term.

Chapter 2

Understanding Your Hormonal Blueprint

To successfully reset your hormones and achieve your weight loss goals, you need to understand how hormones operate uniquely within your body. Each person has a distinct "hormonal blueprint" influenced by genetics, age, lifestyle, and environment. This chapter will help you identify potential hormonal imbalances through self-assessment, recognize the factors affecting your hormone levels, and understand why a personalized approach is key to creating sustainable health changes.

Identifying Hormonal Imbalances: Symptoms and Self-Assessment

Hormonal imbalances manifest in various ways, often as symptoms we might otherwise ignore or attribute to other causes. By tuning into these signs, you can start identifying which hormones may need balancing. Use this self-assessment guide to help spot potential imbalances:

- **Insulin Imbalance**

    Common Symptoms: Constant hunger, cravings for sweets, fatigue after meals, difficulty losing weight, and frequent urination.

    What It Means: If you experience these symptoms, you may have insulin resistance, which leads your body to store more fat, particularly around the abdomen. Managing insulin sensitivity is crucial to improving metabolism and controlling weight.

- **Cortisol Imbalance**

    Common Symptoms: Trouble sleeping, frequent anxiety, low energy, cravings for salty or sugary foods, weight gain around the belly, and mood swings.

What It Means: Chronic stress can keep cortisol elevated, triggering fat storage, especially in the midsection. Balancing cortisol through stress management can lead to better weight control and improved overall health.

- **Thyroid Imbalance**

  Common Symptoms: Unexplained weight gain or difficulty losing weight, fatigue, dry skin, thinning hair, cold intolerance, and depression.

  What It Means: An underactive thyroid slows down metabolism, making it hard to burn calories efficiently. Supporting thyroid health can enhance energy and metabolic rate.

- **Estrogen Imbalance**

    Common Symptoms in Women: Irregular periods, mood swings, bloating, headaches, and weight gain around the hips and thighs.

    Common Symptoms in Men: Low energy, decreased muscle mass, increased body fat, and low libido.

    What It Means: Estrogen imbalances in women can lead to weight gain, particularly around the lower body, while in men, excess estrogen is often linked to increased body fat. Supporting estrogen balance can help manage weight and mood.

- **Leptin and Ghrelin Imbalance**

  Common Symptoms: Constant hunger, cravings even after eating, difficulty feeling full, and an intense desire for high-calorie foods.

  What It Means: When leptin (the hormone that signals fullness) and ghrelin (the hormone that signals hunger) are out of balance, it becomes challenging to control appetite and cravings. Balancing these hormones helps regulate hunger and satiety signals, which is key for weight management.

Encourage readers to keep a journal of their symptoms. Recognizing patterns can help you identify specific areas where you may need to focus in the upcoming chapters.

How Age, Lifestyle, Genetics, and Environment Impact Your Hormone Levels

Hormones are not static—they fluctuate with age, lifestyle choices, genetic predisposition, and even environmental exposures. Understanding how these factors impact your hormones can empower you to make adjustments that support balance.

- **Age**

    In Your 20s and 30s: Hormones like estrogen, testosterone, and growth hormone are typically at their peak. However, poor diet, stress, and lack of sleep can disrupt this balance.

    In Your 40s and 50s: This is a period of hormonal transition for most, with estrogen levels beginning to shift in women (perimenopause) and testosterone levels gradually declining in men. Metabolism may naturally slow down, and maintaining muscle mass and energy levels becomes more challenging.

60s and Beyond: Hormone production continues to decline with age. Both men and women may experience decreased muscle mass, higher body fat percentages, and lowered energy levels. Supporting hormone balance through lifestyle choices becomes even more critical.

- **Lifestyle Choices**

  Diet: A diet high in refined sugars, unhealthy fats, and processed foods can lead to insulin resistance, weight gain, and inflammation—all of which can throw hormones off balance.

Exercise: Physical activity influences hormones like insulin, cortisol, and growth hormone. Different types of exercise have unique effects on hormone health. For example, resistance training helps maintain muscle mass, which is important for metabolic health, especially as we age.

Sleep: Sleep is crucial for hormonal health. Poor sleep disrupts the release of hormones like ghrelin, leptin, and cortisol, leading to cravings, increased appetite, and weight gain.

Stress Management: Chronic stress keeps cortisol elevated, which can cause weight gain around the abdomen and disrupt other hormones like insulin and thyroid hormones. Managing stress through mindfulness, exercise, and relaxation techniques is essential.

- **Genetics**

    Hormonal Predispositions: Genetics play a role in how your body processes hormones. Some people are more sensitive to insulin, while others are more prone to estrogen dominance. Although you can't change your genetics, you can optimize your lifestyle to work with your genetic predispositions.

    Family Health History: Understanding your family's health history can provide clues about potential hormonal challenges you might face. For example, if thyroid issues run in your family, you may be more susceptible to thyroid imbalances.

- **Environmental Factors**

Toxins and Endocrine Disruptors: Exposure to chemicals found in plastics, pesticides, and personal care products can interfere with hormone production and balance. These chemicals, known as endocrine disruptors, mimic hormones and can confuse your body's natural hormone signaling.

Sleep Environment: Factors such as artificial light exposure before bed and lack of darkness during sleep can disrupt the production of melatonin, a hormone that regulates sleep cycles and impacts overall hormonal health.

By understanding how age, lifestyle, genetics, and environment influence your hormones, you can start making conscious choices to support a balanced hormonal state.

Bioindividuality: How Hormonal Health Varies from Person to Person

Just as every person has unique fingerprints, each of us has a unique hormonal makeup shaped by our biology and lifestyle. This concept, known as **bioindividuality**, recognizes that there is no one-size-fits-all approach to hormonal health. Here are some ways bioindividuality comes into play:

- **Metabolic Differences**: Some people metabolize foods and nutrients differently, which can affect blood sugar and insulin levels. While one person may thrive on a lower-carb diet, another may need a balanced approach with moderate carbs to maintain energy and hormonal stability.

- **Stress Response**: Everyone responds to stress differently. Some people have naturally higher baseline cortisol levels, making them more susceptible to stress-related weight gain. Techniques that work well for one person, such as high-intensity exercise, may actually increase stress for someone else with a different cortisol response.

- **Sensitivity to Diet and Toxins**: Certain people are more sensitive to foods or chemicals in the environment. For example, some people have heightened responses to caffeine, which can elevate cortisol and disrupt sleep, while others may not experience these effects.

Recognizing your own bioindividuality allows you to tailor your approach to hormone balancing, focusing on what works best for your body. This personalized approach is essential for long-term success, as it considers your unique needs rather than applying a rigid or standardized protocol.

Chapter Summary and Next Steps
By identifying signs of hormonal imbalances and understanding the factors that influence your hormones, you are now ready to dive deeper into the specific steps needed to create balance. In the following chapters, we'll explore practical strategies to reset each hormone, step-by-step, so you can embrace a healthier, more vibrant body in alignment with your unique hormonal blueprint.

Chapter 3

The Root Causes of Hormonal Imbalance

Hormonal imbalances rarely happen overnight. Often, they are the cumulative result of stress, poor sleep, diet, environmental toxins, and other lifestyle factors that disrupt the body's delicate hormonal balance over time. This chapter explores these common triggers and explains how they can shift your hormones out of balance, leading to weight gain and other health issues. By understanding these root causes, you'll gain insight into how you can begin rebalancing your hormones naturally.

Common Triggers of Hormonal Imbalance

- **Chronic Stress**

    How It Affects Hormones: When you experience stress, your body releases cortisol, the "stress hormone." In small amounts, cortisol is beneficial; it helps you respond to immediate threats. However, chronic stress—whether from work, relationships, or financial pressures—keeps cortisol levels elevated. Over time, high cortisol can lead to insulin resistance, increased appetite, and fat storage, especially around the abdomen.

Signs of Stress-Induced Imbalance: Fatigue, sugar cravings, sleep disturbances, and difficulty losing weight are common signs that chronic stress may be affecting your hormones.

- **Poor Sleep Quality and Irregular Sleep Patterns**

  How It Affects Hormones: Sleep is essential for hormonal balance. During sleep, your body regulates and releases key hormones, including growth hormone, which is essential for muscle repair, fat burning, and overall metabolism. Poor or irregular sleep disrupts the release of these hormones, leading to higher levels of cortisol, reduced insulin sensitivity, and imbalances in hunger hormones like leptin and ghrelin.

Signs of Sleep-Related Imbalance: Waking up tired, experiencing frequent hunger, especially for sugary foods, mood swings, and weight gain, particularly around the midsection, may signal that poor sleep is impacting your hormones.

- **Diet High in Processed Foods and Sugars**

    How It Affects Hormones: Diets high in processed foods and refined sugars lead to frequent spikes in blood sugar, prompting the release of insulin. Over time, constant insulin release can lead to insulin resistance, a condition where cells become less responsive to insulin, leading to fat storage and inflammation. Additionally, unhealthy fats and additives in processed foods can disrupt hormones like estrogen and testosterone.

Signs of Diet-Related Imbalance: Symptoms like constant hunger, sugar cravings, fatigue after meals, and difficulty losing weight, especially around the belly, may indicate diet-related hormone imbalance.

- **Exposure to Environmental Toxins**

    How It Affects Hormones: Many common household products, plastics, pesticides, and even personal care items contain endocrine-disrupting chemicals (EDCs) that mimic or interfere with natural hormones. Chemicals like BPA, phthalates, and parabens can disrupt estrogen, testosterone, and thyroid hormone function. Long-term exposure to these toxins can throw the entire endocrine system off balance.

    Signs of Toxin-Related Imbalance: Weight gain, especially in the hips and thighs, unexplained fatigue, and irregular menstrual cycles (in women) may be signs of hormonal disruption from environmental toxins.

- **Sedentary Lifestyle or Over-Exercising**

  How It Affects Hormones: Physical activity has a profound impact on hormones. Regular exercise can help balance insulin, support thyroid health, and reduce cortisol. However, a sedentary lifestyle can lead to insulin resistance and weight gain, while excessive exercise, particularly intense cardio, can elevate cortisol and disrupt other hormones.

  Signs of Exercise-Related Imbalance: Inactivity can lead to weight gain and sluggishness, while over-exercising can cause fatigue, increased hunger, and difficulty in maintaining a stable weight.

- **Hormonal Changes Due to Aging**

  How It Affects Hormones: Age-related hormonal shifts are natural but can be accelerated or worsened by lifestyle factors. As women approach menopause and men experience declines in testosterone, both sexes may see changes in body composition, energy levels, and metabolism. While we cannot stop aging, lifestyle changes can ease this hormonal transition.

  Signs of Age-Related Imbalance: Gradual weight gain, changes in energy levels, muscle loss, and increased body fat (especially around the midsection) are common indicators of age-related hormonal shifts.

How Lifestyle Factors Disrupt Hormonal Balance and Lead to Weight Gain

Hormones are responsive to daily routines, diet, and stress levels. When these factors fall out of balance, hormone levels are thrown off, creating a domino effect that can lead to weight gain. Let's take a closer look at how this happens:

Blood Sugar and Insulin: When you frequently consume sugary or processed foods, your blood sugar levels spike, causing a surge of insulin to manage it. Repeated spikes in insulin can lead to insulin resistance, a key driver of weight gain, especially around the belly.

Stress and Cortisol: Chronic stress keeps cortisol elevated, which can lead to increased fat storage, particularly in the abdominal area. Elevated cortisol also increases cravings for high-calorie foods, making it challenging to stick to healthy eating.

Sleep and Hunger Hormones: Poor sleep raises levels of ghrelin (the hunger hormone) and reduces levels of leptin (the hormone that signals fullness). This imbalance leads to stronger cravings and less control over appetite, increasing the likelihood of overeating and weight gain.

Environmental Toxins and Estrogen: Exposure to endocrine disruptors in plastics, pesticides, and chemicals can lead to estrogen dominance—a state where estrogen levels are disproportionately high compared to other hormones, leading to fat storage around the hips and thighs. This imbalance can be difficult to address without detoxifying the environment and body.

Physical Inactivity and Metabolic Slowdown: A sedentary lifestyle slows metabolism, reducing the rate at which your body burns calories. Inactivity also contributes to insulin resistance, compounding weight gain and making it harder to lose fat.

The Roadmap to Rebalancing Hormones Naturally

The good news is that hormonal imbalances caused by lifestyle factors can often be reversed or managed through a few simple, natural steps. Here is an overview of the roadmap to balancing hormones naturally, which we'll explore in detail in the following chapters:

Stress Management: Incorporating stress-relief practices such as deep breathing, meditation, and mindfulness can lower cortisol levels and reduce the impact of stress on your hormones. Consistently practicing relaxation techniques is one of the most effective ways to support long-term hormonal balance.

Improving Sleep Quality: Prioritizing sleep hygiene—such as maintaining a consistent sleep schedule, limiting screen time before bed, and creating a calming sleep environment—helps regulate hunger hormones and improve metabolic health. Quality sleep allows your body to reset and restore hormonal balance.

Adopting a Hormone-Friendly Diet: Emphasize whole foods like vegetables, lean proteins, healthy fats, and fiber-rich carbs. This diet helps stabilize blood sugar, support insulin sensitivity, and reduce inflammation. Eating mindfully and including balanced nutrients can help combat cravings and keep hormones in check.

Detoxifying Your Environment: Minimizing exposure to endocrine disruptors in personal care products, food packaging, and household cleaners can help prevent hormonal interference. Opt for natural and organic products when possible and avoid plastics that contain BPA and phthalates.

Incorporating Physical Activity: Aim for a balance between cardio, strength training, and gentle exercises like yoga or walking. Exercise reduces insulin resistance, supports thyroid function, and helps with weight management. Moving regularly and listening to your body's needs can keep your hormones and metabolism steady.

Supporting Digestion and Gut Health: A healthy gut plays a vital role in hormone metabolism and regulation. Incorporate probiotic-rich foods, fiber, and prebiotics to support gut health, which, in turn, supports balanced hormones and reduces inflammation.

Consider Targeted Supplements: Certain supplements, like omega-3 fatty acids, magnesium, and adaptogens, can support hormone balance. However, it's essential to consult a healthcare provider to ensure safe and appropriate supplementation for your needs.

Chapter Summary and Transition
Understanding the root causes of hormonal imbalance empowers you to make proactive changes that support balanced hormones and sustainable weight loss. In the coming chapters, we'll dive deeper into each area, giving you specific, actionable steps to rebalance your hormones naturally and create a healthy, energized body.

Chapter 4

The Nutritional Foundation for Hormonal Health

Nutrition plays a crucial role in balancing hormones and supporting your body's ability to function optimally. Specific nutrients are essential for hormone production, regulation, and overall balance. This chapter will guide you through the basics of a hormone-friendly diet, including foods to prioritize and avoid, and the importance of balancing macronutrients—proteins, fats, and carbohydrates—to maintain hormonal stability.

How Nutrients Support Hormone Production and Balance

Hormones are chemical messengers made from essential nutrients, and without these nutrients, the body struggles to produce and regulate them effectively. Here's a look at key nutrients and how they contribute to hormonal health:

- **Healthy Fats**

  Role in Hormone Production: Hormones, especially steroid hormones like estrogen, progesterone, and testosterone, are derived from fats. Consuming healthy fats ensures your body has the building blocks it needs to create these hormones.

  Sources: Avocados, nuts, seeds, olive oil, coconut oil, and fatty fish like salmon and mackerel provide monounsaturated and omega-3 fats, both essential for hormone health.

- **Protein and Amino Acids**

  Role in Hormone Regulation: Proteins break down into amino acids, which are vital for producing peptide hormones like insulin and growth hormone. Proteins also support tissue repair, immune function, and satiety, helping to maintain stable blood sugar levels.

Sources: Include high-quality protein sources like eggs, lean meats, fish, legumes, and plant-based proteins like tofu and tempeh.

- **Fiber**

  Role in Hormone Balance: Fiber helps regulate blood sugar by slowing digestion and stabilizing insulin levels. It also assists in eliminating excess estrogen from the body through digestion, preventing estrogen dominance and supporting hormonal balance.

Sources: Vegetables, fruits, whole grains, legumes, and nuts are all excellent sources of fiber.

- **Micronutrients**

Zinc: Supports the production of thyroid hormones and is essential for reproductive health. Foods like pumpkin seeds, lentils, and shellfish are rich in zinc.

Magnesium: Known as the "relaxation mineral," magnesium helps lower cortisol, supports insulin sensitivity, and is vital for muscle and nerve function. You can find magnesium in leafy greens, almonds, avocados, and dark chocolate.

Vitamin D: This hormone-like vitamin regulates calcium and is crucial for thyroid health and mood. Vitamin D is found in fatty fish, fortified foods, and can be synthesized from sunlight exposure.

B Vitamins: Essential for energy production and regulating stress hormones, particularly B6 and B12, which support brain and adrenal function. Leafy greens, eggs, and lean meats are great sources.

- **Antioxidants**

  Role in Reducing Inflammation: Hormonal imbalances are often accompanied by inflammation. Antioxidants help reduce inflammation, protecting hormone-producing cells and improving overall hormonal function.

Sources: Colorful fruits and vegetables, like berries, spinach, and bell peppers, along with green tea and spices like turmeric, are rich in antioxidants.

The Hormone-Friendly Diet: What to Eat and What to Avoid

Focusing on nutrient-dense, whole foods can support a healthier hormone balance. Here's a look at the key components of a hormone-friendly diet:

Foods to Eat

- **Leafy Greens and Cruciferous Vegetables**: Kale, broccoli, spinach, and Brussels sprouts are high in fiber and antioxidants, which help detoxify the liver and promote estrogen metabolism.

- **High-Quality Proteins**: Eggs, fish, lean meats, and plant-based proteins provide amino acids that are crucial for hormone production and help stabilize blood sugar.

- **Healthy Fats**: Avocado, nuts, seeds, olive oil, and fatty fish provide essential fats that support hormone synthesis and reduce inflammation.

- **Complex Carbohydrates**: Sweet potatoes, oats, quinoa, and legumes provide fiber and slow-digesting carbs that stabilize blood sugar and insulin levels.

- **Fermented Foods**: Yogurt, sauerkraut, and kefir support gut health, which is critical for hormone balance as the gut microbiome plays a role in metabolizing hormones.

- **Berries and Other Low-Sugar Fruits**: Strawberries, blueberries, and raspberries are high in antioxidants and have a lower glycemic impact, reducing blood sugar spikes that can lead to insulin imbalances.

Foods to Avoid

- **Refined Sugars**: Foods high in sugar can spike insulin levels, contributing to insulin resistance and weight gain. Avoid sodas, candies, and processed foods with added sugars.

- **Processed and Refined Grains**: White bread, pasta, and other refined grains lead to rapid spikes in blood sugar, creating insulin imbalances. Choose whole grains whenever possible.

- **Alcohol and Caffeine**: Both can disrupt hormonal balance, impacting cortisol, estrogen, and testosterone levels. Limit intake, especially if you are sensitive to these substances.

- **Trans Fats and Highly Processed Foods**: Trans fats in fried foods, hydrogenated oils, and ultra-processed snacks contribute to inflammation, which disrupts hormone signaling.

- **Dairy and Soy (for Some)**: Some individuals are sensitive to dairy and soy products, which can impact estrogen levels. If you suspect sensitivity, consider reducing or eliminating these foods.

The Importance of Balancing Macronutrients

Balancing macronutrients (proteins, fats, and carbs) throughout the day can help stabilize blood sugar levels, improve energy, and promote hormone health. Here's a breakdown of each macronutrient's role in hormonal stability:

- **Protein**

  Importance: Protein helps curb hunger and stabilize blood sugar, preventing spikes and crashes that stress the endocrine system. Including protein in each meal keeps energy steady and helps you feel full longer.

  Recommendation: Aim to include a source of protein with every meal, such as eggs at breakfast, lean meat or legumes at lunch, and fish or tofu at dinner.

- **Healthy Fats**

  Importance: Fats are crucial for hormone production, particularly steroid hormones like estrogen and testosterone. Including fats in meals also helps with the absorption of fat-soluble vitamins (A, D, E, K), which are necessary for hormone production and balance.

Recommendation: Include a small serving of healthy fats, such as avocado, olive oil, or nuts, with every meal to support sustained energy and hormone synthesis.

- **Carbohydrates**

  Importance: Carbohydrates provide a quick source of energy and, when paired with fiber, help stabilize blood sugar levels. Complex carbs like whole grains and vegetables contain fiber, which supports digestion and the elimination of excess estrogen.

Recommendation: Focus on fiber-rich carbs such as vegetables, whole grains, and legumes. Aim to avoid refined carbs, which can cause insulin spikes and hormonal imbalance.

Building a Balanced Plate for Hormone Health

Creating balanced meals that include protein, fats, and fiber-rich carbohydrates can help manage blood sugar levels, reduce inflammation, and promote satiety. Here's a simple guide for building a hormone-supportive meal:

- **Fill Half Your Plate with Vegetables**: Aim for a mix of leafy greens and brightly colored veggies. This provides fiber, antioxidants, and essential vitamins.
- **Include a Protein Source**: Choose high-quality protein like chicken, fish, tofu, or

legumes. Protein helps you stay full and supports muscle repair.

- **Add Healthy Fats**: Top your meal with a small serving of avocado, a handful of nuts, or a drizzle of olive oil to support hormone synthesis.

- **Include a Fiber-Rich Carb Source**: Add complex carbs like quinoa, sweet potatoes, or a small portion of whole grains to stabilize blood sugar.

Chapter Summary and Transition
Building a hormone-friendly diet is one of the most effective steps toward long-term hormonal balance. By focusing on nutrient-dense foods, balancing macronutrients, and avoiding processed foods, you can support healthy hormone production, improve metabolism, and feel more energized. In the following chapters, we'll explore

lifestyle practices—such as stress management, sleep improvement, and toxin reduction—that work alongside nutrition to optimize your hormonal health.

Chapter 5

Resetting Your Hormones Through Strategic Eating

Strategic eating patterns can support and reset hormonal balance, particularly when it comes to hormones like insulin, cortisol, and growth hormone. This chapter explores two effective approaches—cyclic eating and intermittent fasting—and how they can impact hormone health and weight loss. With sample meal plans and timing strategies, you'll learn how to tailor your eating patterns to optimize hormone function, boost metabolism, and achieve sustainable weight loss.

Cyclic Eating: Supporting Hormonal Rhythms

Cyclic eating involves adjusting your eating patterns to align with hormonal fluctuations in the body. The concept of cyclic eating fits particularly well with women's hormonal cycles, but men can also benefit from adjusting their food intake to support natural energy and hormone levels throughout the day or week.

- **Cyclic Eating for Women**
  - **Follicular Phase (Days 1–14)**: In the first half of the menstrual cycle (starting from the first day of the period), estrogen levels rise, often resulting in higher energy. During this phase, the body may respond well to more complex carbohydrates, which provide energy for activities and exercise.
    - **Foods to Emphasize**: Whole grains, starchy vegetables, fruits, and lean proteins.
  - **Luteal Phase (Days 15–28)**: During the second half of the cycle, progesterone levels increase, which can slow metabolism and increase cravings. Focus on healthy fats and fiber to manage blood sugar and reduce cravings.

- **Foods to Emphasize**: Healthy fats (avocado, nuts), fiber-rich veggies, and protein-rich foods like eggs and fish.

- **Menstrual Phase (Days 1–5)**: During the menstrual phase, the body may need extra iron and magnesium to replenish what is lost. Comfort foods that are nutritious but gentle on digestion can be beneficial.

  - **Foods to Emphasize**: Leafy greens, lean proteins, magnesium-rich foods (dark chocolate, nuts), and plenty of hydration.

- **Cyclic Eating for Energy and Recovery**

  - For individuals who don't have a menstrual cycle, cyclic eating can still be applied by alternating between higher-carb and higher-fat days to optimize energy and recovery. On active days, slightly increasing complex carbs can fuel activity, while focusing on protein and fat on rest days can support muscle recovery and balance blood sugar.

Intermittent Fasting and Time-Restricted Eating

Intermittent fasting (IF) and time-restricted eating (TRE) have gained popularity as strategies to manage weight and reset metabolic hormones. By limiting the window of time in which you eat, these methods can influence key hormones like insulin, leptin, and cortisol.

- **The Science Behind Intermittent Fasting**
  - **Insulin Sensitivity**: Fasting periods give the body time to lower insulin levels, improving insulin sensitivity. When insulin is kept low, the body is

more likely to tap into stored fat for energy, aiding in weight loss.

- **Growth Hormone Production**: During fasting, growth hormone levels rise, supporting muscle preservation and fat burning.

- **Leptin and Ghrelin Regulation**: Fasting may help reset hunger hormones, making it easier to recognize natural hunger cues and avoid overeating.

- **Popular Intermittent Fasting Methods**

  - **16:8 Method**: Involves fasting for 16 hours and eating within an 8-hour window, which can support a natural circadian rhythm and hormonal balance. For example, eating between 12 pm and 8 pm allows for a morning fasting period that stabilizes blood sugar and reduces late-night eating.

- 5:2 **Method**: Involves eating normally for five days and restricting calorie intake on two non-consecutive days each week. This approach may work well for those who prefer more flexibility.

  - **Alternate-Day Fasting**: This method involves fasting every other day, allowing for more significant fasting periods. However, it can be challenging to sustain and may not be suitable for everyone.

- **Who Should Approach Fasting with Caution**

  - While intermittent fasting can be effective, it's not for everyone. Individuals with a history of disordered eating, certain metabolic conditions, or high-stress levels may find that fasting increases cortisol, leading to stress and hormone imbalance. Women may also need to approach fasting with caution, especially during certain phases of their menstrual cycle, as it can sometimes disrupt hormonal balance.

Sample Meal Plans and Timing Strategies

These sample meal plans incorporate balanced macronutrients and timing strategies to support hormonal health. Adjust the timing based on your chosen intermittent fasting window, if applicable.

- **16:8 Intermittent Fasting Sample Plan**
  - **Fasting Window**: 8 pm–12 pm
  - **Eating Window**: 12 pm–8 pm
  - **Meal Plan**:
    - **12 pm – First Meal**: Spinach and avocado salad with grilled salmon, quinoa, and a drizzle of olive oil. Include a side of berries for antioxidants.

- **3 pm – Snack**: Greek yogurt with a sprinkle of chia seeds and sliced almonds.
- **6 pm – Dinner**: Grilled chicken breast with roasted sweet potatoes and steamed broccoli, topped with a handful of walnuts.
- **8 pm – Light Snack (Optional)**: Sliced cucumber and bell peppers with hummus, if needed.

- **Cyclic Eating Sample Plan for Women (by Phase)**
  - **Follicular Phase** (Higher Carb)
    - **Breakfast**: Overnight oats with chia seeds, berries, and a dollop of almond butter.
    - **Lunch**: Lentil and vegetable stir-fry with brown rice.

- **Dinner**: Grilled shrimp with a side of roasted carrots, sweet potatoes, and steamed spinach.

- **Luteal Phase** (Higher Fat and Protein)

  - **Breakfast**: Scrambled eggs with sautéed greens and avocado.

  - **Lunch**: Tuna salad with mixed greens, olives, cucumber, and olive oil.

  - **Dinner**: Baked salmon with roasted cauliflower and Brussels sprouts.

- **Menstrual Phase** (Iron-Rich)

  - **Breakfast**: Smoothie with spinach, banana, chia seeds, almond milk, and a spoonful of cacao powder.

  - **Lunch**: Chickpea and roasted beet salad with pumpkin seeds.

- **Dinner**: Grass-fed beef stir-fry with peppers, broccoli, and quinoa.

- **Balanced Plate Sample for Non-Cyclers or Beginners**
    - **Breakfast (8 am)**: Greek yogurt with mixed berries, a handful of walnuts, and chia seeds for fiber and healthy fats.
    - **Lunch (12 pm)**: Grilled chicken with a leafy green salad, cherry tomatoes, a small portion of quinoa, and a drizzle of olive oil.
    - **Afternoon Snack (3 pm)**: Apple slices with almond butter or a small handful of nuts.
    - **Dinner (6 pm)**: Baked cod with steamed asparagus, roasted butternut squash, and a side salad.

Timing Strategies to Support Weight Loss and Hormone Optimization

- **Eat During Daylight Hours**: Eating during daylight helps align your eating patterns with your circadian rhythm, which can improve insulin sensitivity and reduce cortisol spikes from late-night meals.

- **Don't Skip Breakfast (If Needed)**: While fasting can be effective, some people benefit from a protein-rich breakfast. If you find that skipping breakfast increases stress, try having a high-protein, low-carb breakfast to stabilize blood sugar.

- **Include Protein with Every Meal**: Protein reduces blood sugar spikes, making it essential at each meal to support steady energy and prevent insulin imbalances.

- **Limit Late-Night Eating**: Eating late in the evening can increase insulin levels at night, which may interfere with fat-burning.

Finish your last meal at least two to three hours before bed to allow insulin levels to drop.

Chapter Summary and Transition Strategic eating patterns like cyclic eating and intermittent fasting can reset hormones, improve insulin sensitivity, and support healthy weight loss. By aligning your meals with your body's natural rhythms, you create an environment for optimal hormone function. In the next chapter, we'll explore stress management techniques to further support your journey toward balanced hormones and improved well-being.

Chapter 6

Managing Stress and Balancing Cortisol

Stress has a powerful influence on hormone health, especially through its impact on cortisol, the body's primary stress hormone. When cortisol levels are consistently elevated, it can disrupt other hormones and contribute to weight gain, particularly around the abdomen. In this chapter, we'll explore cortisol's role in the body, why chronic stress can lead to weight gain, and practical techniques for reducing stress and restoring hormonal balance. Self-care practices and a strong mind-body connection are also essential tools for fostering hormonal health and overall well-being.

Understanding Cortisol's Role in the Body and Weight Gain

Cortisol is produced by the adrenal glands and released in response to stress. It plays an important role in helping the body manage energy by mobilizing glucose for quick fuel. However, when stress becomes chronic, so does cortisol production, which can lead to a host of hormonal and metabolic issues, including weight gain.

- **How Cortisol Contributes to Weight Gain**
  - **Abdominal Fat Accumulation**: Cortisol promotes fat storage, especially around the abdomen, as a protective mechanism for energy reserves during times of stress. Abdominal fat cells also contain more cortisol receptors, making them especially sensitive to high levels of this hormone.
  - **Increased Hunger and Sugar Cravings**: Chronic stress often leads to elevated cortisol and adrenaline levels, which can increase appetite and cravings for high-sugar or high-fat "comfort foods." This cycle can disrupt blood sugar and insulin

levels, leading to further hormonal imbalance.

- o **Disrupted Sleep**: Cortisol follows a natural rhythm, rising in the morning to help you wake up and dropping in the evening to prepare for sleep. Chronic stress can disrupt this cycle, leading to poor sleep quality and even higher cortisol levels, which exacerbates weight gain.

- **The Cortisol-Insulin Connection**
  - o Cortisol and insulin are closely linked; when cortisol remains elevated, it can increase insulin levels, leading to insulin resistance. This reduces the body's ability to process glucose, causing blood sugar spikes and increasing the risk of fat storage.

Techniques for Reducing Stress and Balancing Cortisol

Bringing cortisol back into balance requires managing both the sources of stress and the body's response to it. Here are several effective techniques for managing stress and balancing cortisol:

- **Mindfulness and Meditation**
    - **Mindfulness**: Practicing mindfulness—focusing on the present moment without judgment—can significantly reduce cortisol levels and ease stress. Simple techniques, like mindful breathing or body scanning, encourage you to observe and release tension.
    - **Meditation**: Regular meditation has been shown to reduce cortisol, promote relaxation, and improve emotional resilience. Even just 5-10

minutes a day of meditation can have profound benefits for cortisol levels and overall stress reduction.

- o **Guided Practices**: Consider using apps or online resources for guided meditation and mindfulness sessions. Options like body scan meditation or guided imagery can be especially helpful for stress reduction.

- **Breathing Exercises**

  - o **Diaphragmatic Breathing**: Also known as deep belly breathing, this technique involves taking slow, deep breaths that engage the diaphragm. Diaphragmatic breathing has been shown to lower cortisol and shift the body into a more relaxed state.

  - o **Box Breathing**: Box breathing, or four-square breathing, involves inhaling for a count of four, holding for four, exhaling for four, and holding again for four. This structured breathing pattern calms the nervous system and can quickly reduce stress.

- o **Practice**: Start by finding a quiet space, inhaling deeply through the nose, filling your belly with air, holding briefly, and then exhaling slowly. Repeat for a few minutes to feel more grounded and relaxed.

- **Physical Activity and Movement**

  - o **Gentle Exercise**: Activities like yoga, tai chi, and walking can help reduce cortisol without overtaxing the body. These types of exercise promote relaxation and help balance stress hormones without triggering an additional cortisol response, which can happen with high-intensity workouts.

- **Yoga and Stretching**: Yoga, in particular, combines mindful movement with breathing techniques, helping to reduce cortisol, improve flexibility, and promote a sense of calm. Yin yoga, which involves holding poses for longer periods, can be especially beneficial for stress relief.
  - **Daily Movement**: Even simple activities, like a daily walk in nature or gentle stretching at home, can help reduce stress, improve circulation, and lower cortisol levels.

- **Sleep Hygiene**
  - **Regular Sleep Routine**: A consistent sleep schedule can help restore natural cortisol rhythms. Going to bed and waking up at the same time each day supports

circadian rhythm and improves sleep quality.

- o **Create a Relaxing Bedtime Routine**: Engage in calming activities before bed, such as reading, stretching, or taking a warm bath. Avoid screens, caffeine, and heavy meals close to bedtime to promote a more restful sleep environment.

- o **Magnesium Supplementation**: Magnesium, the "relaxation mineral," can promote better sleep and reduce cortisol. Consider incorporating magnesium-rich foods or a magnesium supplement before bed, if appropriate.

- **Connection and Social Support**

  - o **Social Connection**: Spending time with friends, family, or even pets can help reduce cortisol by fostering feelings of safety and support.

Positive interactions release oxytocin, a hormone that counteracts cortisol and promotes relaxation.

- **Setting Boundaries**: Prioritizing your well-being sometimes means saying no to additional commitments. Establish boundaries that allow you to manage stress more effectively, reducing feelings of overwhelm.

- **Community Activities**: Participating in community events or joining support groups can provide an outlet for stress and help you feel less isolated, which can lower cortisol and improve resilience.

The Importance of Self-Care and the Mind-Body Connection

Self-care and a strong mind-body connection are essential for maintaining balanced cortisol levels and supporting hormone health. Taking time for yourself and actively engaging in relaxation practices reinforces to your body that it is safe and doesn't need to stay in "fight or flight" mode. Here are some ways to incorporate self-care into your routine for lasting benefits:

- **Prioritize "Me Time"**
  - Dedicate a few minutes each day to activities that bring you joy and relaxation. Whether it's reading, crafting, or spending time in nature, prioritizing these moments helps your body understand it doesn't need to stay in a stressed state.,

- **Practice Gratitude**

  - Taking time each day to reflect on things you're grateful for has been shown to reduce stress and improve mood. Gratitude practices can shift focus away from stressors and create a more positive outlook, which reduces cortisol over time.

- **Body Awareness Techniques**

  - Practices like progressive muscle relaxation and body scanning help increase body awareness, allowing you to notice and release physical tension. By tuning in to how stress manifests in your body, you can work to release it through mindful relaxation techniques.

- **Nourishing Your Body with Self-Care Foods**

  - Certain foods can help support stress resilience. Foods high in antioxidants (like berries), omega-3s (like salmon and walnuts), and B vitamins (found in leafy greens) support brain health and stress reduction.

- o Herbal teas, like chamomile or lemon balm, can also provide relaxation benefits. Drinking a warm cup of tea can become a calming self-care ritual that signals to your body it's time to unwind.

Chapter Summary and Transition

Balancing cortisol is key to overall hormonal health and successful weight management. Chronic stress and elevated cortisol can lead to weight gain, especially around the midsection, and disrupt other hormones critical for health. By practicing regular stress reduction techniques like mindfulness, breathing exercises, and prioritizing self-care, you can bring cortisol back into balance. With consistent effort, these practices not only help control cortisol but also promote a sense of well-being, supporting a balanced, healthy life.

Chapter 7

The Role of Sleep in Hormone and Weight Management

Sleep is a cornerstone of health, impacting everything from brain function to immune strength. Yet, it is often overlooked when it comes to weight management and hormone balance. Research shows that poor sleep can disrupt critical hormones that control appetite, metabolism, and stress responses, leading to weight gain and hormone imbalances. This chapter dives into how sleep influences these key hormones, offers practical strategies for improving sleep quality, and shares tips for creating a sleep-friendly environment and routine.

How Sleep Affects Hormones and Weight

During sleep, your body undergoes essential repair and regulatory processes. A lack of quality sleep can throw off hormone balance, particularly in hormones related to appetite and metabolism, making weight management much more challenging.

- **Ghrelin and Leptin: Hormones of Hunger and Satiety**

  o **Ghrelin**: Known as the "hunger hormone," ghrelin signals to your brain that it's time to eat. When you're sleep-deprived, ghrelin levels increase, often leading to heightened hunger and cravings for high-calorie foods.

  o **Leptin**: Leptin is the "satiety hormone" that signals fullness and helps regulate energy balance. Insufficient sleep decreases leptin levels, making it harder for you to feel satisfied after meals, leading to overeating and weight gain.

  o **The Ghrelin-Leptin Imbalance**: Sleep deprivation creates a hormonal imbalance by boosting ghrelin and lowering leptin, which can lead to an increased appetite and cravings, particularly for sugary, high-fat foods.

- **Insulin Sensitivity and Blood Sugar Control**
  - Poor sleep can lead to reduced insulin sensitivity, meaning the body becomes less efficient at using glucose for energy. When insulin sensitivity is impaired, blood sugar levels stay elevated, which can increase fat storage, especially around the abdomen. Chronic poor sleep can even increase the risk of insulin resistance, a precursor to metabolic conditions like diabetes and obesity.

- **Cortisol and Stress Response**
  - Sleep is essential for maintaining healthy cortisol levels. With insufficient or poor-quality sleep, cortisol levels may remain elevated,

triggering a chronic stress response that encourages fat storage and muscle breakdown. This can lead to weight gain, particularly in the midsection, and contribute to a vicious cycle of poor sleep and elevated cortisol.

- **Growth Hormone and Muscle Repair**
  - Growth hormone is primarily released during deep sleep and plays a crucial role in muscle repair, fat burning, and metabolism. Without enough deep sleep, growth hormone production decreases, leading to muscle loss and a slower metabolism.

Strategies for Improving Sleep Quality

Improving sleep quality requires adopting habits that support your body's natural sleep rhythms. Here are practical strategies to help you get the restorative sleep you need to support hormone health and weight management:

- **Establish a Consistent Sleep Schedule**
  - Going to bed and waking up at the same time every day reinforces your body's circadian rhythm. Aim for at least 7-8 hours of sleep per night, and try to stick to your schedule, even on weekends. This consistency helps regulate cortisol and melatonin (the sleep hormone), making it easier to fall asleep and wake up naturally.
- **Optimize Your Pre-Sleep Routine**
  - **Wind Down**: Engage in relaxing activities in the hour leading up to bedtime. Gentle stretching, reading a book, or practicing mindfulness meditation can signal to your body that it's time to prepare for sleep.

o **Limit Stimulants**: Avoid caffeine and nicotine in the late afternoon and evening, as these stimulants can stay in your system for hours, making it harder to fall asleep. Additionally, consider limiting alcohol close to bedtime, as it can disrupt sleep quality.

o **Avoid Late-Night Meals**: Try to finish eating at least 2-3 hours before bed. Late-night eating can increase blood sugar and insulin levels, potentially interfering with the body's natural overnight repair processes.

- **Manage Light Exposure**

o **Natural Light During the Day**: Exposure to natural light in the morning helps regulate your circadian rhythm, promoting better sleep. Try to get outside for a few minutes each morning, even if it's cloudy, to reinforce your body's internal clock.

- o **Limit Blue Light in the Evening**: Blue light from screens (phones, computers, TVs) interferes with melatonin production, making it harder to fall asleep. Consider using blue light filters on devices or avoiding screens for at least an hour before bed. Instead, opt for relaxing activities that don't involve screens.

- **Exercise Regularly**
  - o Regular physical activity can improve sleep quality, reduce stress, and enhance overall well-being. However, avoid vigorous exercise close to bedtime, as it can increase cortisol and adrenaline, making it harder to wind down. Try to

complete intense workouts at least a few hours before bed.

Creating a Sleep-Friendly Environment

Your bedroom environment can significantly influence your ability to fall asleep and stay asleep. By making a few adjustments, you can create a space that promotes restful, uninterrupted sleep.

- **Keep Your Bedroom Cool, Dark, and Quiet**
    - **Cool Temperature**: The ideal bedroom temperature for sleep is typically around 65°F (18°C). A cooler environment helps lower core body temperature, which is essential for initiating sleep.
    - **Block Out Light**: Use blackout curtains or an eye mask to create a dark environment. Darkness signals

to your brain that it's time to sleep by stimulating melatonin production.

- o **Reduce Noise**: Use earplugs or a white noise machine if you're in a noisy area. Consistent background noise can help mask disruptive sounds and improve sleep continuity.

- **Invest in Comfortable Bedding**
  - o **Mattress and Pillows**: Choose a mattress and pillows that provide proper support and comfort. Investing in high-quality bedding can make a big difference in your sleep quality, as discomfort from poor bedding can lead to frequent wake-ups and restless sleep.
  - o **Breathable Fabrics**: Use breathable, natural materials for your sheets and blankets. Cotton or bamboo fabrics are generally comfortable choices

that help regulate body temperature throughout the night.

* **Remove Distractions and Keep Your Bedroom for Rest**

   o **Limit Electronics**: Keeping TVs, phones, and other electronics out of the bedroom creates a space dedicated to rest and relaxation. If you need an alarm clock, opt for a simple one rather than relying on your phone.

   o **Create a Calming Atmosphere**: Add elements that promote relaxation, such as calming scents (lavender or chamomile essential oils), soft lighting, or gentle music. These additions can signal to your brain that the bedroom is a place for rest.

Practical Tips for Building a Healthy Sleep Routine

A healthy sleep routine can improve both the quality and duration of your sleep. Here are some tips for cultivating sleep-friendly habits:

- **Start a Pre-Sleep Relaxation Routine**
    - Establish a consistent wind-down routine each night to signal to your body that it's time to sleep. This might include a warm bath, a few minutes of journaling, or reading a book. Over time, your body will come to associate these activities with preparing for sleep.

- **Limit Fluids in the Evening**
    - Drinking too much fluid close to bedtime can lead to frequent bathroom trips, disrupting sleep. Try to hydrate adequately throughout the

day and limit fluid intake in the hours leading up to bedtime.

- **Consider Natural Sleep Aids**
    - **Herbal Teas**: Chamomile, valerian root, and passionflower teas can promote relaxation and support sleep.
    - **Magnesium**: This essential mineral helps calm the nervous system and may promote better sleep quality. You can take magnesium in supplement form or through foods like leafy greens, almonds, and pumpkin seeds.
    - **Melatonin Supplements**: In some cases, a low-dose melatonin supplement can help regulate sleep cycles, especially if you experience occasional disruptions. However,

consult a healthcare professional before using melatonin or any sleep aid.

Chapter Summary and Transition

Sleep is a foundational component of hormone and weight management, influencing everything from appetite-regulating hormones like ghrelin and leptin to stress-related hormones like cortisol. By prioritizing sleep hygiene and creating a sleep-friendly environment, you set yourself up for better hormone balance, improved energy, and more effective weight management. In the next chapter, we'll explore how physical activity can further support hormonal health and aid in sustainable weight loss.

Chapter 8

Movement and Hormones: The Right Exercise for You

Exercise is a powerful tool for supporting hormone balance and promoting weight loss, but not all types of movement affect hormones in the same way. While intense exercise can stimulate hormones like cortisol and adrenaline, gentler movement supports relaxation and stress relief. In this chapter, we'll explore how different forms of exercise—strength training, cardio, high-intensity interval training (HIIT), and gentle movements—impact hormones and metabolism. By understanding the unique effects of each type of movement, you'll be able to choose the exercise routine that best supports your body and your goals.

How Different Types of Exercise Affect Hormones

Each type of exercise engages the body differently, influencing specific hormones that control metabolism, appetite, stress, and even sleep. Here's how some popular exercise styles impact hormone levels:

- **Strength Training**
  - **Hormones Impacted**: Testosterone, growth hormone, and insulin sensitivity.
  - **Benefits**: Strength training, or resistance training, builds lean muscle mass, which is essential for a healthy metabolism and fat burning. This type of exercise promotes the release of testosterone and growth hormone, both of which play key roles in muscle repair and fat loss. Strength training also increases insulin sensitivity, helping the body manage blood sugar more efficiently.
  - **Weight Loss and Hormones**: By boosting lean muscle, strength training increases your resting

metabolic rate, meaning you burn more calories even at rest. This makes it an ideal form of exercise for long-term weight management.

- **Cardiovascular Exercise (Cardio)**
  - **Hormones Impacted**: Endorphins, cortisol (when excessive), and insulin sensitivity.
  - **Benefits**: Cardiovascular exercise includes activities like running, cycling, swimming, or brisk walking. It improves heart health, increases endurance, and releases endorphins—the "feel-good" hormones that help reduce stress and improve mood. Regular cardio can also enhance insulin sensitivity, supporting healthy blood sugar levels.
  - **Weight Loss and Hormones**: While cardio is effective for calorie burning

and improving cardiovascular health, excessive cardio can raise cortisol levels, which may actually interfere with weight loss goals. For hormone health, balance moderate cardio with other forms of exercise.

- **High-Intensity Interval Training (HIIT)**
  - **Hormones Impacted**: Human growth hormone (HGH), testosterone, and insulin.
  - **Benefits**: HIIT combines short bursts of intense exercise with brief recovery periods. This form of exercise triggers a strong release of growth hormone and testosterone, which supports fat burning and muscle repair. HIIT also boosts insulin sensitivity, helping manage blood sugar.
  - **Weight Loss and Hormones**: HIIT is efficient for weight loss because it

maximizes calorie burn in a short amount of time and promotes an "afterburn" effect, where your body continues to burn calories post-workout. However, it should be done in moderation to avoid cortisol spikes.

- **Gentle Movements (Yoga, Pilates, Walking)**
    - o **Hormones Impacted**: Cortisol, serotonin, and endorphins.
    - o **Benefits**: Gentle movements like yoga, Pilates, and walking are excellent for reducing stress and balancing cortisol levels. These forms of exercise improve flexibility, reduce tension, and enhance relaxation without overstimulating stress hormones. Yoga, in particular, is known to increase serotonin, the

"happy hormone," promoting a sense of calm.

- **Weight Loss and Hormones**: While gentle movements may not burn as many calories as intense workouts, they play a critical role in stress management and cortisol control, which is essential for sustainable weight loss and hormonal health.

Choosing the Right Exercise Regimen for Hormonal Health and Weight Loss

When it comes to exercise, balance is key. Here are guidelines to help you choose the right exercise plan for optimizing hormone balance and supporting weight loss:

- **Prioritize Strength Training for Metabolism and Muscle Health**
  - Aim for 2-3 sessions of strength training per week. Focus on

compound movements, like squats, lunges, deadlifts, and push-ups, which engage multiple muscle groups and maximize calorie burn. By building muscle, you'll boost your metabolism and enhance insulin sensitivity, both of which contribute to effective weight loss.

- **Incorporate Cardio for Heart Health and Endorphins**

  o Cardio is beneficial for cardiovascular health and can help with weight loss when done in moderation. Aim for 2-3 cardio sessions per week, focusing on moderate-intensity activities like jogging, cycling, or brisk walking. Limit long-duration cardio sessions to prevent excessive cortisol release, which can work against your hormonal balance and weight loss efforts.

- **Add HIIT for Efficient Calorie Burn**
  - If you're short on time, incorporate HIIT sessions 1-2 times per week. HIIT can effectively burn calories and stimulate hormones that support muscle growth and fat loss. However, because HIIT is intense, keep sessions brief (around 20-30 minutes) and allow for adequate recovery between workouts.

- **Embrace Gentle Movement for Stress Relief and Cortisol Control**
  - To counterbalance more intense workouts, integrate gentle movements like yoga, stretching, or walking into your routine. Aim for 2-3 sessions per week, or even daily if possible. These activities promote relaxation and improve sleep,

supporting cortisol regulation and overall hormonal health.

Sample Workout Plans to Support Hormone Balance and Weight Loss

Here are three sample workout plans that combine different types of exercise to support hormone health, metabolism, and sustainable weight loss. Adjust these plans to fit your fitness level and schedule.

- **Sample Plan 1: Balanced Routine for Overall Hormone Health**
  - **Day 1**: Strength Training (full-body)
  - **Day 2**: Moderate-Intensity Cardio (30 minutes jogging or cycling)
  - **Day 3**: Gentle Movement (yoga or 30-minute walk)
  - **Day 4**: HIIT (20-minute session)
  - **Day 5**: Strength Training (upper body focus)

- **Day 6**: Gentle Movement (Pilates or stretching)
- **Day 7**: Rest or Gentle Movement (easy walk)

- **Sample Plan 2: Stress Relief and Cortisol Management**
  - **Day 1**: Moderate Cardio (30 minutes walking or swimming)
  - **Day 2**: Gentle Yoga or Pilates
  - **Day 3**: Strength Training (lower body focus)
  - **Day 4**: Gentle Movement (30-minute walk)
  - **Day 5**: Strength Training (upper body focus)
  - **Day 6**: Rest or Meditation
  - **Day 7**: Moderate Cardio or Gentle Movement (low-intensity cycling or hiking)

- **Sample Plan 3: Fat-Burning and Muscle-Building Routine**

- Day 1: Strength Training (full body with compound exercises)
  - **Day 1**: Strength Training (full body with compound exercises)
  - **Day 2**: HIIT (20-25 minutes)
  - **Day 3**: Gentle Yoga or Rest
  - **Day 4**: Strength Training (lower body focus)
  - **Day 5**: Moderate Cardio (30-minute jog)
  - **Day 6**: HIIT or Strength Training (upper body focus)
  - **Day 7**: Rest or Gentle Movement (stretching or easy walk)

Tips for Staying Consistent with Exercise for Hormone Health

- **Listen to Your Body**
  - Pay attention to how your body responds to different forms of exercise. If you feel overly fatigued or stressed, incorporate more gentle

movement and rest days to keep cortisol levels balanced.

- **Prioritize Rest and Recovery**
  - Rest days are essential for hormone balance, especially after intense workouts. Adequate recovery helps prevent overtraining, which can elevate cortisol and disrupt other hormones. Aim for at least one rest day per week and consider incorporating stretching or light yoga on these days.

- **Set Realistic Goals**
  - Choose goals that focus on how exercise makes you feel rather than only on appearance or weight loss. Setting achievable goals like improving strength, increasing flexibility, or enjoying stress relief can help you stay consistent with your exercise routine.

- **Stay Flexible**

  - ○ Life can be unpredictable, so be willing to adapt your workout schedule as needed. Remember, it's the consistency that counts, not perfection. Find joy in movement, and focus on progress rather than perfection.

Chapter Summary and Transition

Exercise plays a crucial role in balancing hormones and supporting weight management. By incorporating a combination of strength training, cardio, HIIT, and gentle movements, you can create a well-rounded routine that enhances your metabolism, improves your mood, and helps you manage stress. In the next chapter, we'll explore the importance of mindful eating, which complements your exercise routine by helping you tune into your body's needs and signals.

Chapter 9

Detoxifying Your Life for Hormonal Balance

Our bodies are constantly exposed to environmental toxins and chemicals that can disrupt hormone function, contributing to imbalances that impact everything from weight to mood. In this chapter, we'll explore how these toxins, including endocrine disruptors, affect hormonal health. You'll also find practical strategies to reduce exposure to these chemicals and support your body's natural detoxification pathways to improve overall hormonal balance.

The Impact of Environmental Toxins on Hormone Health

Endocrine disruptors are chemicals that can interfere with hormone systems, potentially causing a range of health issues. Found in common products like plastics, pesticides, and personal care items, these chemicals can mimic or block hormones and throw off our body's natural balance. Some common endocrine disruptors include:

- **Bisphenol A (BPA)**: Found in plastics and food can linings, BPA can mimic estrogen in the body, which may contribute to weight gain, reproductive issues, and increased estrogen dominance.

- **Phthalates**: Used in fragrances, plastics, and cosmetics, phthalates can interfere with testosterone production and affect reproductive health.

- **Parabens**: Common preservatives in cosmetics and personal care products, parabens can mimic estrogen and disrupt hormone function.

- **Pesticides**: Chemicals in conventional farming practices can act as endocrine disruptors and affect hormone balance, especially thyroid function.

- **Heavy Metals (e.g., lead, mercury)**: These metals can accumulate in the body over time and interfere with hormone production and metabolism, particularly impacting thyroid health and adrenal function.

When we accumulate toxins in our body, it can overburden our liver, which plays a critical role in processing and excreting excess hormones and detoxifying harmful substances. By supporting liver function and reducing toxin exposure, we can enhance hormone balance and support sustainable weight management.

Tips for Reducing Toxin Exposure in Daily Life

- **Choose Organic and Non-Toxic Foods**
  - Whenever possible, choose organic produce, which is grown without synthetic pesticides and herbicides. This is especially important for fruits and vegetables that are commonly sprayed with pesticides, like strawberries, spinach, and apples. Consider the "Dirty Dozen" and

"Clean Fifteen" lists as guides for prioritizing organic foods to reduce pesticide exposure.

- o Avoid processed foods that often contain artificial ingredients, preservatives, and additives that can disrupt hormones. Look for whole, minimally processed foods that nourish the body and support hormone health.

- **Switch to Natural Skincare and Personal Care Products**

  - o Many conventional personal care products contain endocrine-disrupting chemicals like parabens, phthalates, and synthetic fragrances. Switch to products with natural, organic ingredients free from harmful chemicals.

  - o For skincare, look for "fragrance-free" products or those scented with natural essential oils. Additionally, check labels for ingredients like sodium lauryl sulfate (SLS) and synthetic colors, which can irritate the skin and burden the body with unnecessary toxins.

- **Use Safe Cooking Utensils and Containers**
    - Plastic containers can leach chemicals, especially when heated, so opt for glass or stainless steel containers for food storage. Avoid microwaving food in plastic containers, as the heat can increase the leaching of chemicals like BPA and phthalates into food.
    - Choose non-toxic cookware, such as ceramic or stainless steel, rather than non-stick cookware, which often contains perfluorinated chemicals

(PFCs) linked to hormone disruption and other health risks.

- **Create a Cleaner Home Environment**
  - Use natural cleaning products to avoid exposure to harmful chemicals found in many conventional cleaners. Simple ingredients like vinegar, baking soda, and essential oils can effectively clean surfaces without introducing toxins.
  - Ventilate your home regularly to reduce indoor air pollution. Adding air-purifying plants, like spider plants or peace lilies, can also help to filter toxins and improve air quality.

- **Reduce Exposure to Heavy Metals**
  - Limit exposure to heavy metals by choosing fish low in mercury, such as salmon, sardines, and trout. If you consume fish frequently, consider avoiding larger fish, like swordfish or

tuna, which tend to have higher mercury levels.

- o Use a water filter to remove heavy metals and other contaminants from drinking water. Look for filters that specifically target lead, chlorine, and other impurities.

A Gentle Detox Plan to Support Liver Function and Hormone Processing

Supporting your liver's natural detoxification processes can help the body clear out excess hormones and environmental toxins, promoting a more balanced hormonal system. Below is a gentle detox plan that focuses on nourishing the liver without extreme restrictions or harsh methods.

- **Hydrate with Lemon Water**
  - o Start your day with a glass of warm water and a squeeze of fresh lemon. This helps stimulate digestion,

supports hydration, and encourages liver function. Throughout the day, aim to drink plenty of water to help flush toxins from the body.

- **Incorporate Liver-Supportive Foods**
  - Certain foods are known to support liver health and detoxification, including:
    - **Cruciferous Vegetables**: Broccoli, cauliflower, and Brussels sprouts contain compounds that help activate liver enzymes responsible for detoxifying toxins and excess hormones.
    - **Leafy Greens**: Spinach, kale, and chard are rich in chlorophyll, which helps cleanse the blood and support liver function.

- **Beets and Carrots**: These vegetables contain beta-carotene and plant compounds that promote liver health and aid in hormone processing.

- **Garlic and Onions**: Rich in sulfur, these allium vegetables support liver detoxification and hormone balance.

- **Try an Herbal Liver Support Blend**

  - Herbal teas or supplements containing milk thistle, dandelion root, and turmeric can provide extra support for liver detoxification. These herbs promote liver health, reduce inflammation, and support the breakdown of toxins. Speak with a healthcare provider before adding any new supplements to your routine.

- **Increase Fiber Intake**

    o Fiber-rich foods, such as oats, chia seeds, flaxseeds, and whole grains, bind to toxins in the digestive system and help escort them out of the body. Fiber also helps to prevent the reabsorption of excess hormones in the gut, promoting a healthy balance.

- **Limit Alcohol and Caffeine**

    o Both alcohol and caffeine can place additional stress on the liver, impacting its ability to process hormones effectively. Reducing your intake or incorporating alcohol-free days can support liver health and reduce inflammation, improving overall hormonal balance.

- **Prioritize Sleep and Restorative Practices**

    o Sleep is essential for detoxification, as the liver and other organs work to process toxins during rest. Aim for 7-9 hours of quality sleep per night and include restorative practices, like gentle yoga or meditation, to reduce stress and support adrenal health.

Practical Tips for a Toxin-Reduced Lifestyle

- **Practice Mindful Consumption**
  - Try to adopt a "less is more" approach to personal care and cleaning products. Often, using fewer products that are more natural can reduce the body's toxic burden significantly.

- **Detoxify at Your Own Pace**
  - You don't need to make all these changes at once. Begin with small steps, such as switching out one household product or incorporating one liver-supportive food into your

diet. Over time, these changes add up to create a healthier, hormone-friendly environment.

- **Listen to Your Body**
    - o As you reduce toxin exposure and incorporate gentle detox practices, pay attention to how your body feels. You may notice improvements in energy, mood, and even weight, as your hormones begin to rebalance.

Chapter Summary and Transition

Toxins are all around us, but with practical lifestyle changes, you can reduce your exposure and support your body's natural detox pathways. By nourishing your liver and choosing hormone-friendly products, you'll be taking an important step toward achieving balance and sustainable weight management. In the next chapter, we'll look at the importance of mental and emotional well-being for long-term hormone health, exploring the impact of mindfulness, emotional resilience, and self-care practices.

Chapter 10

Supportive Supplements for Hormonal Health

While a balanced diet and healthy lifestyle are foundational for hormonal health, certain supplements can play a supportive role in rebalancing and optimizing hormone function. In this chapter, we'll explore some of the most effective supplements for hormone health, from essential nutrients to adaptogens. You'll also learn how to choose high-quality supplements, use them safely, and understand when it might be beneficial to consult a healthcare provider before starting a new supplement.

The Role of Supplements in Hormonal Balance

Supplements can offer targeted support for specific hormones and processes, providing the body with nutrients that might be missing or in low supply. For instance, some people may have difficulty getting enough omega-3 fatty acids or magnesium through diet alone, and targeted supplementation can fill these gaps. When used thoughtfully, supplements can aid in reducing symptoms, promoting stability, and supporting the body's natural hormonal cycles.

Key Supplements for Hormone Balance

- **Omega-3 Fatty Acids**
  - **Benefits**: Omega-3s, commonly found in fish oil, have powerful anti-inflammatory properties that support overall hormonal health, brain function, and heart health. They play a role in managing cortisol and can help stabilize mood and reduce inflammation, which is crucial for balancing hormones.
  - **Sources**: Omega-3s are found in fatty fish like salmon and sardines. For those who prefer plant-based options, flaxseed, chia seeds, and walnuts are good sources, though they provide a less potent form of omega-3s.

- o **Dosage**: Look for supplements containing EPA and DHA, ideally from a reputable fish oil source. Typical doses range from 1,000 to 3,000 mg per day, but always follow product recommendations.

- **Magnesium**
  - o **Benefits**: Magnesium is often called the "relaxation mineral" because it's essential for stress management, muscle relaxation, and sleep quality. It supports adrenal function and can help lower cortisol levels, making it especially beneficial for those dealing with stress-related hormone imbalances.
  - o **Sources**: Magnesium is abundant in leafy greens, nuts, seeds, and whole grains, but many people still fall short of their daily needs.

- o **Forms and Dosage**: Magnesium glycinate and magnesium citrate are two easily absorbed forms. A typical dosage ranges from 200-400 mg per day, often taken in the evening to support sleep.

- **Adaptogens (e.g., Ashwagandha, Rhodiola, Maca)**
  - o **Benefits**: Adaptogens are herbs that help the body adapt to stress, regulate cortisol, and support overall hormonal balance. Ashwagandha, for example, is known for its ability to reduce stress and improve adrenal health. Rhodiola can help increase energy and resilience, while Maca is particularly beneficial for balancing sex hormones.
  - o **Usage**: Adaptogens are generally taken in capsule, powder, or tea form. Each adaptogen has its own unique

properties, so start with one and note any changes in mood, energy, or stress levels.

- o **Dosage**: Follow the product's instructions for dosing, as dosages can vary significantly depending on the form and concentration of the adaptogen.

- **Vitamin D**

  - o **Benefits**: Vitamin D functions more like a hormone than a vitamin and is critical for many bodily functions, including hormone production, immune function, and mood regulation. Low vitamin D levels are associated with hormonal imbalances, especially related to thyroid and sex hormones.

  - o **Sources**: Sun exposure is the best source of vitamin D, but it's also found in fortified foods and supplements.

- o **Dosage**: Dosages can vary depending on current levels; many people benefit from 1,000-5,000 IU per day. It's wise to get your levels tested and consult with a healthcare provider to determine the appropriate dosage.

- **B Vitamins (especially B6, B12, and Folate)**

  - o **Benefits**: B vitamins play a key role in energy production, brain health, and the synthesis of neurotransmitters, which affect mood and stress response. Vitamin B6 is essential for estrogen metabolism, while B12 and folate are crucial for cellular energy and adrenal health.

  - o **Sources**: B vitamins are found in animal products, leafy greens, and fortified grains. Those with dietary restrictions (e.g., vegetarians or vegans) may be more likely to need supplementation.

- o **Dosage**: Look for a high-quality B-complex supplement that provides a range of B vitamins. Dosages can vary, but B6 is commonly taken at 10-50 mg per day and B12 at 500-1,000 mcg per day.

- **Probiotics**

  - o **Benefits**: The gut microbiome plays a critical role in hormone balance, particularly in estrogen metabolism and cortisol management. Probiotics support a healthy gut environment, aiding in digestion, nutrient absorption, and immune function.

  - o **Sources**: Fermented foods like yogurt, kefir, sauerkraut, and kimchi are natural sources of probiotics, though supplementing can be beneficial for more targeted support.

- **Dosage**: Probiotic supplements vary widely, but a typical range is 1-10 billion CFUs (colony-forming units) per day. Choose a multi-strain formula for broader benefits.

- **Zinc**

  - **Benefits**: Zinc is essential for reproductive health and immune function, playing a vital role in hormone synthesis and balancing testosterone levels. Zinc also supports thyroid function and can improve insulin sensitivity, which is important for weight management and hormonal stability.

  - **Sources**: Zinc is found in foods like oysters, beef, pumpkin seeds, and chickpeas. Supplementing can be beneficial for those with low dietary intake or absorption issues.

- o **Dosage**: Zinc dosages typically range from 15-30 mg per day, but consult a healthcare provider if taking higher amounts, as too much zinc can interfere with copper balance.

Guidelines for Safe Supplement Use

- **Choose High-Quality Supplements**
  - o Look for reputable brands that use third-party testing to verify purity, potency, and safety. Supplements marked with certifications such as NSF, USP, or GMP indicate higher quality standards.
- **Start Low and Monitor Your Response**
  - o When introducing a new supplement, start with a lower dose to see how your body reacts, especially with

herbs and adaptogens. Pay attention to any physical changes, mood shifts, or energy levels, and adjust as needed.

- **Be Consistent**
  - Supplements generally work best when taken consistently over time. Establish a routine that allows you to take your supplements regularly and track your progress.

- **Consider Bioavailability**
  - Some nutrients, such as magnesium and vitamin B12, come in forms that are more or less absorbable by the body. Look for "bioavailable" forms, which are easier for your body to absorb and use, maximizing the benefits.

- **Avoid Over-Supplementing**
  - More isn't always better. Overuse of certain supplements, like vitamin D

or zinc, can have adverse effects. Always stick to recommended dosages unless advised otherwise by a healthcare professional.

When to Consult a Healthcare Provider

Although many supplements are safe and beneficial, certain health conditions, medications, or individual sensitivities may require special consideration. You may want to consult with a healthcare provider if you:

- Are pregnant, breastfeeding, or planning to become pregnant.
- Have a chronic health condition, such as diabetes, thyroid disorder, or autoimmune disease.
- Are currently taking prescription medications, as some supplements can interact with certain drugs.

- Experience adverse reactions to a supplement or find that your symptoms worsen.

- Are unsure of your nutrient levels and would like to test for deficiencies (e.g., vitamin D, magnesium, or iron).

Chapter Summary and Transition

Supplements can be a powerful addition to your hormone-balancing journey, offering targeted support where you need it most. By choosing the right supplements and using them mindfully, you can work toward greater hormonal balance, enhanced energy, and improved weight management. In the next chapter, we'll focus on putting all these elements together into a holistic, personalized plan to support your unique hormonal needs and help you achieve lasting results.

Chapter 11

Tracking Progress and Adjusting for Long-Term Success

The journey to hormonal health and weight management is a dynamic process that goes beyond the numbers on a scale. In this chapter, we'll explore effective ways to track progress in a holistic way, recognizing changes in energy levels, mood, physical measurements, and overall well-being. We'll also discuss how to make adjustments to your routine as your needs evolve and provide strategies for sustaining these lifestyle changes to avoid common setbacks.

Redefining Progress: It's More Than Just Weight

While weight can be one marker of progress, it doesn't fully capture improvements in hormone health or overall wellness. A successful journey involves tracking multiple aspects of health, allowing you to see the broader impact of your efforts. Here are a few important markers of progress:

- **Energy Levels**

    o Improvements in hormone balance often correlate with increased energy and vitality. Notice how your energy fluctuates throughout the day. Are you feeling more awake in the morning? Less fatigued in the afternoon? Keep an energy journal to track your ups and downs and celebrate days when you feel your best.

- **Mood and Emotional Well-being**

    o Hormones influence mood, anxiety levels, and resilience to stress. Reflect on your emotional health: Are you feeling more balanced, less irritable, or calmer under stress? Journaling or using a mood-tracking app can be a great way to monitor emotional progress.

- **Physical Measurements and Body Composition**
  - Instead of relying solely on weight, consider tracking measurements around your waist, hips, and thighs. Body composition, such as muscle tone and fat distribution, is a more accurate measure of physical changes than weight alone, especially as you engage in exercise that builds muscle.

- **Sleep Quality**
  - As hormones come into balance, sleep should improve, helping you wake up refreshed and energized. Keep track of your sleep patterns, noting both duration and quality. A good night's sleep is a strong indicator that your efforts are having a positive impact.
  -

- **Digestive Health**
  - Balanced hormones contribute to better digestive function. If you're experiencing fewer symptoms like bloating, gas, or constipation, it's a sign that your body is responding well to the dietary and lifestyle adjustments you've made.
- **Menstrual Cycle Regularity** (for women)
  - If you've been working on balancing hormones related to the menstrual cycle, regularity and reduced PMS symptoms are significant indicators of progress. A consistent cycle, with manageable symptoms, is a positive sign of hormonal health.

Tools for Tracking Your Progress

To make tracking as simple and effective as possible, here are some tools that can help you monitor changes:

- **Journaling**: Writing down observations about your mood, energy, and sleep each day can offer valuable insights over time.

- **Apps**: There are several health-tracking apps for tracking energy, sleep, and mood patterns, allowing you to view trends and make connections between different factors.

- **Measurements and Photos**: Monthly measurements and progress photos can reveal physical changes that aren't always visible day-to-day. They're particularly useful for seeing body composition changes, such as increased muscle tone or decreased bloating.

- **Symptom Tracker**: A simple chart or checklist for tracking symptoms like headaches, fatigue, or digestive discomfort can highlight improvements that may otherwise go unnoticed.

Adjusting Your Plan for Long-Term Success

Hormonal balance is not a one-size-fits-all goal, and over time, your body's needs will shift based on factors like age, lifestyle, and stress levels. Learning to adapt your plan as needed is essential for sustainable success.

- **Listening to Your Body**
  - Tuning into how you feel is key. If your energy starts to dip, or you're experiencing new symptoms, it may be time to re-evaluate aspects of your diet, exercise, or stress management routines. Trusting your body's

signals will help you stay aligned with what it needs.

- **Making Seasonal Adjustments**
  - Hormonal health can benefit from seasonal eating and lifestyle changes. For example, in winter, focusing on warming foods and gentle, restorative exercise can support metabolism and immune function. In the summer, lighter meals and more outdoor activities may feel natural and supportive.

- **Reassessing Nutrition and Supplement Needs**
  - Your nutritional needs may shift as your hormones stabilize. After a few months, consider revisiting your supplement routine to see if adjustments are needed. You might find that you no longer need certain

supplements or that new ones could be beneficial.

- **Adjusting Your Exercise Routine**
  - As your fitness and energy levels improve, you might feel ready to increase the intensity or try new types of exercise. Always listen to how your body responds; if you feel overly fatigued or sore, consider scaling back and focusing on rest.

- **Revisiting Stress-Reduction Techniques**
  - Periods of higher stress may require additional focus on relaxation practices like meditation, yoga, or even taking extra rest days. Re-evaluate your stress management strategies and don't hesitate to try new methods if you need a change.

Sustaining Lifestyle Changes: Tips for Avoiding Common Setbacks

Long-term success with hormone balance is about creating a lifestyle that feels natural and enjoyable rather than restrictive. Here are some tips for maintaining your progress and avoiding common setbacks:

- **Create Routines You Enjoy**
  - Habits are easier to sustain when you genuinely enjoy them. Choose exercises you look forward to, cook foods you love, and find stress-relief practices that feel relaxing and meaningful to you.
- **Plan Ahead for Busy Times**
  - Life's demands can disrupt routines, so having a plan can make a difference. Prepare healthy snacks, meal prep, and keep some quick,

nutritious options on hand to avoid falling back into old habits during busy periods.

- **Celebrate Small Wins**

  - Acknowledging progress in any form—whether it's improved energy, better sleep, or a positive mood—keeps you motivated. Take time to appreciate these shifts as signs that your body is responding well to your efforts.

- **Cultivate a Growth Mindset**

  - Long-term change requires a flexible, open mindset. Instead of seeing setbacks as failures, view them as learning opportunities. Reflect on what caused a lapse in routine and adjust as needed without guilt.

- **Find Support and Community**
  - Having people around who share similar goals can be a great source of motivation and accountability. Whether it's family, friends, or an online community, connecting with others who support your journey can help you stay committed.
- **Revisit Your Goals Regularly**
  - Your goals may evolve as your body and needs change. Reassess your intentions periodically to ensure that your plan aligns with what you truly want, whether it's maintaining energy, improving mood, or achieving further physical changes.

Chapter Summary and Final Thoughts

Tracking progress through diverse markers beyond the scale helps you celebrate and recognize improvements in energy, mood, sleep, and overall well-being. Adjusting your plan as life changes ensures you stay in harmony with your body's needs, creating a sustainable path to health. By setting up supportive routines and adapting with flexibility, you're not only working toward balanced hormones but also creating a lifestyle that supports your well-being for years to come.

As you continue this journey, remember that hormone health is a long-term commitment to yourself and your vitality. Trust in your body's ability to heal and adapt, and know that every small effort contributes to the lasting results you're building.

Chapter 12

Your New Life: Embracing a Balanced and Healthy Body

As you reach the final chapter of this journey, it's time to look back at the transformations you've achieved, the tools you've gained, and the positive changes in how you feel, look, and think about health. Building a life that supports balanced hormones and a healthy weight is more than a goal—it's a way of living that nurtures your mind, body, and spirit every day.

In this closing chapter, we'll reflect on the steps you've taken, celebrate the progress you've made, and inspire you to embrace this lifestyle for the long term. This journey is now yours to continue and personalize, empowering you to live a vibrant, fulfilling life that prioritizes your well-being.

Reflecting on the Journey

Achieving hormonal balance is no small feat, and your progress is a testament to your dedication, resilience, and commitment to change. You've taken intentional steps to learn about your body, understand the power of hormones, and adopt habits that support a healthier, happier life. Consider all you've gained:

- **A Deeper Understanding of Your Body**: You've explored the powerful ways hormones impact weight, mood, energy, and overall health. With this knowledge, you're now better equipped to recognize the signs of imbalance and know how to respond with care and insight.

- **Lifestyle Changes That Support Hormonal Health**: From dietary adjustments and mindful movement to stress reduction and quality sleep, you've integrated practices that go beyond weight loss. These changes support your body's natural rhythms and promote resilience in the face of life's demands.

- **Tools for Resilience and Adaptability**: Hormonal health is not about rigid rules or quick fixes—it's about adaptability, tuning in to your body's needs, and knowing how to adjust your routines to stay aligned with your health goals.

Embracing a Lifestyle That Prioritizes Hormonal Health

As you move forward, embracing this balanced lifestyle is about committing to wellness in all areas of life. Here are a few guiding principles to carry with you:

- **Make Well-Being a Priority, Not a Task**
  - Think of wellness as something that enhances your life, not as an obligation. A balanced approach means making healthy choices that bring you joy, energy, and satisfaction, rather than forcing yourself into routines that feel restrictive or stressful.

- **Listen to Your Body and Trust Its Signals**
  - Your body is an amazing communicator. When you feel low on energy, out of sync, or moody, it's often a sign that your hormones may need attention. Use what you've learned to fine-tune your routine based on these cues. Small adjustments, like improving sleep or rebalancing nutrients, can make a huge difference.
- **Stay Curious and Open to Change**
  - The journey doesn't end here. As your body changes with age, lifestyle shifts, or new life circumstances, your hormonal needs may shift too. Staying open and adaptable allows you to evolve with your body and make choices that support you at every stage.

- **Celebrate Progress Over Perfection**

    o Embracing a balanced lifestyle doesn't mean every day will be flawless. There will be days when things don't go as planned, and that's perfectly fine. Celebrate the overall progress you've made, and remember that consistency over time is far more valuable than perfection.

- **Honor the Connection Between Body and Mind**

    o Your mental and emotional well-being is closely tied to your hormonal health. Keep prioritizing practices that promote inner calm, self-compassion, and resilience, whether through mindfulness, meditation, or simply taking time each day to relax and recharge.

Final Thoughts: A Sustainable Approach to Health

The tools and insights you've gained are part of a lasting lifestyle transformation. Rather than focusing on rigid goals, this approach encourages you to see health as a dynamic, evolving process. Prioritizing balance, listening to your body, and adapting to life's changes will create a foundation that supports your health for years to come.

Hormonal health is deeply intertwined with overall well-being. By committing to a lifestyle that nurtures both your physical and mental health, you're giving yourself the gift of vitality, longevity, and resilience. Remember that you are in control of your health journey, and you have the power to make choices that honor and support your body's needs.

Embracing Your New Life

As you step into this new chapter, reflect on how far you've come and embrace the empowerment that comes from understanding your body. Maintaining hormonal balance isn't just about weight management; it's about creating a life filled with energy, happiness, and well-being.

Take each day as an opportunity to reinforce the healthy habits you've established, to continue learning and evolving, and to celebrate the positive impact your choices have on your life. Here's to a future where your hormones are balanced, your energy is strong, and you feel deeply connected to a life of wellness.

Thank you for allowing me to guide you on this journey. May this be the beginning of a lifetime of health, happiness, and harmony. Embrace your new life with confidence, gratitude, and excitement for all the good things to come.

About Jasmin Brooks

Jasmin Brooks is passionate about helping others achieve lasting health and wellness. After her own journey through the ups and downs of weight loss, she realized that the key to success lies in sustainable habits, not quick fixes. In *Forever Fit: Lose Weight and Keep It Off for Good*, Jasmin shares her personal experiences and valuable insights, providing readers with practical tools and a clear, no-nonsense approach to reaching their fitness goals. Her mission is to save you time and frustration by delivering only the most effective strategies for lifelong health.